Sexual Gymnastics

Intimate Fitness

How to Use Ben Wa Balls

Perfume With Pheromones

Girls Have their Own Secrets

Gloria Westwood

Table of Contents

Book Description

Just a few simple tips and you will easily become more confident and sexy. Experience that highest sense of pleasure and gain self-confidence. Surprise your partner and take care of your woman health.

Little secrets of unlimited sexual possibilities – all that your woman happiness offers.

Introduction

Want to talk with you on an intimate topic, which is generally considered to be private. Well, who we talk to about this? Maybe to a friend? Well, it's like loudly shouting at the window, many people can hear that. However, if you are lucky no one will really do. With your mom and sister? Well, probably yes, and that's pretty much all. I was planning to write on this long time ago but every time I kept postponing this. No, I won't call myself a person who blushes from the word "sex" ... in fact, I can easily talk on any topic and today I will be fairly frank. I'm not going to use synonyms, I will call a spade a spade instead, and so shy girls you would feel probably a little uncomfortable. Sorry.

I recommend everyone to try diversifying their world of sensations and orgasm. Yes to sex, yes to sex with toys and dirty movies. But not always we are so super sexy and young. I want to write about keeping myself in a great shape, or rather, keeping my intimate places in a great shape. This is not only pleasant but also useful. Elastic and resilient vaginal muscles make the delivery less painful and positively contribute to your woman health. Even more, the trained vaginal muscles are more important than any other muscle for women's health. However, the lovely ladies, you need to balance things do not be lazy and do not overdo it, you are not going to crack nuts with this part of your body, and it's good to keep your boyfriend safe, and not to screw the meaning of his life.

During making love, a woman and a man can experience incredible feelings as a result of a tight grip of the penis inside the vagina. Well, this can be with any gender though (not necessarily with a male); in any case, the feeling is just super.

Often time's young ladies complain about problems in relationships, lack of interest in sexual intimacy, attitude to sex as to conjugal duties, anorgasmia - and have no idea how to change their sexual life and stop dreaming about the pleasures that are written in women's novels. Women after 30 years, especially if they have children, can already experience the unpleasant consequences of stretched and weak perineal muscles, such as the lowering of the walls of the vagina, bladder, and uterus. So, the best solution is to start working on the Kegel system or head to a sex shop after the postpartum period. And it is even better to pick something from the exercises, add vaginal balls to it and finally take care of beloved yourself.

And you: Cannot get the desired pleasure from sex? Do not feel excited? Tips from magazines do not help to become a skillful mistress? Has sex become a conjugal duty?

Are you having a hard time in your relationships? Do you spend the night alone or not able to find your favorite shoulder in the morning? If the above applies to you - then read on very carefully!

All this can be corrected by Kegel exercises or Ben Wa balls. So, let's compare what will be the effect of the balls and Kegel exercises. Balls and other simulators train the muscles along the entire length, Kegel only trains the muscles of the entrance, and inside he leaves the so-called "dips" - untrained muscles. For the same reason, I can not call Kegel's exercises an absolute helper.

Kegel Training

First, We Will Assess the State of Our Muscles

- We put a finger in the vagina and try to squeeze it, the muscles of the vagina should wrap around the finger just like a ring. The extent to which this ring grabbed the finger is exactly the condition of your muscles. Another way... while urinating, delay this process and stop the flow, then continue, then hold again ...can you make this happen? - perfect, while you do this you should try to not move your legs and your breathing should be calm, in case it does not work - don't worry, the exercises will fix it. If you did not get distracted by lovely yourself, which is just fine, let's keep reading further.

Kegel exercises are the most well-known training method for increasing the tone of the pelvic floor muscles, which supports the uterus, bladder, rectum and small intestine. This technique was developed and described by well-known 20th-century gynecologist Arnold Kegel. Later this group of pelvic floor muscles began to be called "Kegel's muscles". Muscles of the pelvic floor are almost not involved in everyday life, so over time (especially - after childbirth), they lose their elasticity. This can lead to the state when the muscles simply stop coping with their main function - maintaining the pelvic organs. This can lead to various diseases, as well as to the deterioration of sexual life. But these problems can be avoided by regularly performing a set of exercises.

Preparing for Exercise

Before you begin to perform Kegel exercises, you should empty your bladder. These exercises can be done sitting, lying or standing - in any position. To achieve a worthwhile effect you need to exercise 3-4 times a day, 5-40 times per set. It is not recommended to drastically exceed the given number of exercises, as this can only aggravate the problem, from which you will get the opposite effect.

Compression is the basic movement of all Kegel exercises. It is quite simple to understand what muscles you need to train and constantly squeeze: they can be felt during the urination pause.

How to perform Kegel exercises at home.

While performing Kegel exercises, avoid straining other muscle groups - buttocks, thighs, or abdominal cavity. During each exercise, you need to breathe and in no case, you should hold your breath. This will help to relax and achieve the best results (most women see the results after 4-6 weeks).

Block of Five Kegel exercises

1. Exercise "Hold"

Contract the pelvic floor muscles for 5-10 seconds, and then relax. Repeat 10 times per set four times a day and gradually increase the number of repetitions to 50 four times a day.

2. Exercise "Contracting"

Rhythmically contract the pelvic floor muscles for 5 seconds, then relax them and rest for 5 seconds. Do 3-5 sets of 10 repetitions. Gradually increase the duration of the muscle retention time to 10 seconds.

3. Exercise "Elevator"

Imagine that you are in an elevator, which constantly keeps moving up and down. Begin to strain the muscles of the pelvic floor and increase the strength of tension when lifting the elevator higher and higher. When you reach the uppermost floor, smoothly relax the muscles, pausing on each floor and imagining that the elevator returns to the first floor. Then take a trip to the basement where your pelvic floor muscles are completely relaxed.

4. Exercise "Waves"

In this exercise, not only the muscles of the vagina will be involved, but also the muscles of the anus. To perform it, you need to contract the muscles of your vagina, then your anus, and in the same order to relax them. Contractions can reach a duration of 10-20 seconds.

5. Exercise "Positioning"

This exercise is very effective for pregnant women. Before doing it, be sure to pre-clean the intestines. Relax, hold your breath, then extinguish a little, like when emptying. You can try doing this exercise in different positions - lying, sitting, squatting or on all fours. Also, doctors recommend combining this exercise with respiratory gymnastics.

Do everything smoothly, as if you hold the most precious treasure inside you.

Ben Wa Balls

If you want to make a man always see in you a goddess and to feel like a goddess yourself, to turn your sex life into an uninterrupted firework of emotions and omissions. Increase sensitivity and self-confidence. You need to try the Ben Wa balls. What are the Ben Wa balls? They are products designed to strengthen the walls of the vagina, some of them can be used for pleasure. It is enough to go to any sex shop or online store to understand how they look: separate or stitched together, most often with a loop on the end. They are made of a wide variety of materials, can be of various shapes, diameters, weights, have a flat or embossed surface - in short, for every taste and of any color.

Balls are the most ancient vaginal simulator, their analogs have been used since long time ago and they are still loved by many women for their usability and tremendous effect.

They were an invention used in ancient China by geishas to train their own sexuality. But they have not lost relevance in a contemporary world, so today they are widely used by women not only to train the internal muscles of the genital organs but also to diversify their sexual lives. Ben Wa balls are usually made of latex, silicone, glass, metal, and plastic. The configuration is oval or rounded. Balls are often equipped with relief bends in the form of ribs or pimples.

Why do we need Ben Wa balls? We need them to strengthen the muscles of the pelvic floor. Despite the widespread opinion, vaginal balls are not recommended for use as sex toys. And why should your partner know this little secret? Just let him think that you are such a super sexy woman by nature (which is absolutely true by the way).

Vibrating products, the so-called "vibro eggs" are the exceptions though. Classic balls are designed to strengthen the muscles of the pelvic floor, especially those that surround the vagina, narrowing or widening its lumen. Why develop muscles, the existence of which we often do not notice in everyday life?

It turns out that the pelvic diaphragm plays an important role in the life of each person. Even more, it's of particular importance for women. Muscles and ligaments of the small pelvis are exposed to many negative effects throughout life, such as pregnancy; childbirth; frequent lifting of weights; hormonal changes (especially during menopause); passive lifestyle; partial muscle atrophy, occurring with age.

Classic balls are connected by a cord and have a loop, so it is convenient to pull them. Some models have an elastic bond between the balls. The number of balls varies from one to five.

Balls with vibration have a wired or wireless control panel. Balls can be heavy and with a shifted center of gravity. The latter is designed for the beginners who have recently started exercising vaginal muscles.

Weighted balls, as a rule, are made of metal and are designed to maintain the result and enhance the effect. Only girls with developed and powerful muscles of the vagina can cope with them. Ben Wa balls with vibration can provide lots of excitement, so they are preferable to use in sex games as a sex toy for fomenting desire or during an intimate foreplay.

Girls often opt for large and medium-sized balls, believing that the use of large and heavy balls will be more effective. But this is not entirely true. You need to start with balls of small weight and large diameter, constantly increasing the mass and reducing the size. The truth is that the smaller the balls, the more force the muscles will need to move them inside the vagina. What results can a woman achieve by mastering the technique of using Ben Wa balls? Developed and trained muscles of the vagina provide unlimited potential, which allows a female to regulate the diameter of the vagina by squeezing and expanding it.

Daily exercises with balls help a woman to study the anatomy of her body, to know her own sexual feelings and help to get extra pleasure.

In addition, they increase the flow of blood into the pelvic area, which has a favorable effect on the erotic perception of women and allows you to overcome frigidity and anorgasmia.

Every woman should know how to use Ben Wa balls. A special role is played by Ben Wa balls in the process of restoring the female body after childbirth, in order to return the diameter of the vagina to the dimensions that used to be before the birth.

Due to the unique massaging, that occurs during exercises with Ben Wa balls, the inflow of blood to the deep vaginal areas, which are not stimulated during sex, doubles, as a result of which the possibility of blood stasis decreases.

It is also important that training with the use of Ben Wa balls develops the muscles of the genitourinary system, as well as the entire hip area. And maintaining this area in tone is not only the basis of sexual life but also necessary for the functioning of all important female organs. That is why doctors often prescribe Ben Wa balls as a preventive measure against blood stasis.

Before embarking on the use Ben Wa balls must be thoroughly washed and treated with an antiseptic (you can take a lubricant based on miramistine or chlorhexidine). Further, to ensure a comfortable and painless insertion of the balls, it is also recommended to use an intimate lubricant - moisturizing, for example.

Ben Wa balls are best inserted in the position of lying or reclining, to ensure easy penetration into the vagina. It is important to relax as much as possible and listen to your feelings. First enter one, after ten seconds the second. Lie down, listen to your feelings and let the balls properly settle. The free edge of the thread connecting the balls must be left outside so that it will be possible to remove the balls from the vagina.

Next, you can start doing the exercises, and after the training, you have to take out the balls, relax your muscles, wash them thoroughly with warm water and soap and put them in a case.

It is important to use Ben Wa balls with moderation and regularity. The best way is to do it for ten minutes every day instead of one-hour exercise once a week.

Ben Wa Balls Exercises

1 Exercise

One of the simplest exercises is keeping the balls inside. To do this, the balls need to be inserted into the vagina and you need to try to keep them with your muscles for 1-2 minutes. Time can be gradually increased to half an hour, based on your desire and the capabilities of your body.

2 Exercise

The next exercise is walking with balls. It can already be started after a couple of days after the first exercise when the feeling of strength of muscles appears. Movement with vaginal balls inside provides a massage effect, which leads to the reduction in the muscles of the vagina and the saturation of its walls with blood.

3 Exercise

When holding balls and walking with them is already mastered, you can try to manipulate them by moving the balls up and down and from side to side with the help of vaginal muscles.

4 Exercise

The next exercise is pushing and resistance. You should try to push the balls out one by one with the help of vaginal muscles, without helping with fingers or a thread. You can also pull the string, and the muscles of the vagina while trying not to let the balls out.

Further on, to consolidate the results obtained and improve skills, you can perform the same exercises using balls of smaller diameter but with more weight. The question of whether vaginal balls can be used during sex or with vibrators is surely a natural one. Experts strongly recommend retaining from this, but if you really want, it's better to prefer special balls of smaller size that are ideally suited for sexual games.

By the way, vaginal balls cannot be used for anal stimulation as their design is not adapted for painless and easy removal from the anus. For this purpose, it is recommended to use anal stimulants.

Although Ben Wa balls are a toy for sex and stimulation, they are not allowed for women suffering from infectious or inflammatory diseases of the reproductive system. Women who are inclined to allergies should also consult a doctor before using such balls. Do not do this during your period.

Do not be shy! Try and experiment.

From the History

For a long time, secrets on the use of Ben Wa balls were stored in the palace of the emperors, and only empresses and concubines of emperors were able to use them. Many of those who mastered this technique had very good health, keeping in their old age the same resilient and full of love bodies that they had when they were young unmarried girls.

The art of controlling the body arose in ancient times. Chinese, Japanese, Indonesian and later on followed by Greek and Roman sexual masters all used special exercises and adaptations for the development of these important intimate muscles. Very rich Chinese, who were able to maintain a harem, actively encouraged their wives to use a variety of simulators. The most effective stone simulator was the one in the form of an egg.

For a long time, the secrets of using the vaginal balls of Ben-Wa (in China they are called Mienlin) were kept in the palace of the emperors, and only empresses and concubines of emperors were able to use them.

In ancient India, two round-shaped stones used to get inserted into the young girls' vaginas in order to train their vaginal muscles. In Japan, these were two balls of metal or ivory. Young ladies were forced to keep these items in themselves, and under no circumstances to let them fall out. This game of muscles was a special art in India, and the brides who were able to do it were highly valued, and a large ransom was required for them. Japanese geishas kept this art for enthusiastic suitors and special receptions only. Improved, more modern beads were brought from the Far East to the land of freedom France in the 18th century. The French called them pommes d`amour (apple of love) and used this fruit of enjoyment both in palaces to create a kind of frivolous furors, and in the best houses.

My dear ladies, even in the turmoil of days, you can and should devote yourself some time. If you do household chores, you can do it with Ben Wa balls or dance your favorite song with them. Absolutely tired? Do Kegel exercises when brushing your teeth. You can perform exercises almost anywhere - while driving a car, walking, watching TV, sitting at a table, lying in bed. At the beginning of the session, it may turn out that your muscles do not want to remain tense during slow contractions. You may not be able to perform the contractions fast enough or rhythmically. This is because the muscles are still weak. Control improves with practice. If the muscles are tired in the middle of the exercise, rest for a few seconds and continue. Perhaps at some point, you will understand that everything is already narrow and wonderful, so you do not need these balls and exercises anymore. Oh, probably a lot of women would envy you.

But all this improves and creates harmony with your body, feelings are strengthened, the frequency of orgasms increases. Gentlemen, maybe I will destroy someone's dream world now. But yes, we do not often experience the vaginal orgasm, and some of us experience it in very, very rare cases. Do not be selfish, study your woman, talk to her about it, be frank. This applies to ladies too - this is your favorite person and these are your relationships.

In conclusion, I want to say that Kegel's exercises are very effective, I have been trying them on a regular basis for six months already and the results please both me and my husband. I deliberately kept silent and waited for his opinion, but based on certain things I understood that he really liked it and had new pleasant feelings. A week later, he said, "What's going on with you? You're doing something unusual."

When the pelvic area is straining, the whole complex of perineal muscles starts working, including those on which hemorrhoids can arise. During the exercise, blood circulation improves, and there is no stagnation in the veins. Not surprisingly, this complex is now recommended not only to women but also to men. A strong half of humanity also often suffers from hemorrhoids and Kegel exercises help to solve some other problems too.

Be healthy, and sexually happy!

Perfume With Pheromones

Well, every woman has her own secrets, and I want to share some with you.

And I want to write, about the secret weapon of allurement... About perfume with pheromones.

Pheromones are special hormones that are responsible for the attractiveness and sexiness of a person in the eyes of the opposite sex.

I got acquainted with these fragrances through advertising. One pharmacy in my city was running an advertising campaign of perfumes with pheromones. As a part of the campaign, you were allowed to turn the bottle in your hands, smell the various flavors. They also had neutral ones, so that you could use your favorite fragrances and pheromones without mixing the scents. You even could test the fragrance on yourself.

I put on some of the flavors I liked, and then went on my business ... Actually, I did not plan to buy them ... Well, I did not exactly until my husband felt the fragrance!

As soon as I got into the car my husband felt something new. Did your violent imagination draw a scene, where he pounces at me in a fit of passion???

Oh no, this did not happen! However, I was amazed to the fact that he generally paid attention to perfume. He usually never cared about the perfume I was using, and here you are! He even praised it!

Well, I made a conclusion that the pheromones worked. They are must have!

No, I was not going to allure all men. I have a beloved husband, with whom we have been together for more than ten years. But, you know, still, you want to somehow stir up the subsided passion. And I must say that I did not have to use anything extraordinary it was just pheromones and they did their job. They perfectly coped with their task. However, I was always skeptical about them until I tried it myself and witnessed the result.

Let's Talk About them in More Detail:

Perfume with pheromones. What are pheromones, how were fragrances created with them? How do perfumes with pheromones work, how to apply them correctly, what are their characteristics and where they can be bought?

The incredible power of odors is an established fact. Unknowingly, people are looking for their loved ones by the way of being attracted by their smell. Each person has his/her own odor. That's why you are usually able to find exactly the person who can be called your second half in a random crowd.

But science does not stand still. Over time, new ways of deceiving the nature keep popping up. With plain pheromones perfume, a person acquires a specific smell, which can only be caught at the level of instincts.

The creators of these fragrances report that their product is capable of attracting many more potential lovers to the possessor. Just a few drops of perfume are enough to attract the attention of the best people of the opposite sex and get their love. But is it really true that perfumes with pheromones help to become irresistible in the eyes of opposite sex? Or it is just a beautiful fairy tale?

In order to understand how these fragrances act, you first need to understand how they differ from all the others.

Pheromones are special chemicals that are produced in the body of each person. Their function is to attract the opposite sex and to light a desire in them. Pheromones do not guarantee a long and happy love, but they are good in awakening sexual attraction. Do not confuse it with other feelings. It is also necessary to remain cautious. Some people do not know how to control their desires.

Pheromones are produced in the armpits and, surprisingly, in the zone of nose and lips. However, nowadays it is much more difficult for them to perform their natural functions. Every year, a large number of cosmetics are produced, which help disguise our natural smell and cover it with another, artificial one. Although it smells good, it can not attract the opposite sex. It is not like pheromones that are produced by the human body.

Creating Perfume With Pheromones

Science enters into all spheres of human life. The relationship between the sexes is not an exception. For scientists, the main mystery remained the question of what the love actually is? Why does a woman like a particular man, and not the other one, and vice versa? And then pheromones were discovered.

For the first time, perfumes with pheromones appeared not so long ago, in 1989. The birthplace of this novelty can be considered the United States, it was there that for the first time fragrances appeared on the shelves. And they immediately caused both a huge amount of criticism and positive reviews.

Some people have thought about the ethical side of the issue. They believed that people do not have the right to interfere in nature and make their own adjustments to what should be natural. Others did not tired of repeating that, thanks to this novelty, they began to enjoy immense popularity among the opposite sex. And some buyers being disappointed reported that the fragrance made absolutely no change.

Since then, the production of perfumes with pheromones has spread throughout the world. Now it is much easier to find them and they cost much less than they used to. Many countries now have their local companies producing this kind of perfume. The only problem is to pick the one that seems to be the most reliable.

Features of Perfume With Pheromones

Although the creators of fragrances say that their products will help in attracting every one of the opposite sex, you should not blindly believe them. The thing is that human pheromones are still a mystery to scientists. It is absolutely certain that they exist. But we still fail in accurately detecting and recreating them. So don't think that the fragrances with pheromones have the same effect as the natural human body produced pheromones have.

There is always a risk that the producer will sell you a simple perfume instead of advertised pheromones. This way, an expensive bottle can turn out to be a plain fragrant water.

But perfumes with pheromones won't be completely useless in any case. Lady who bought a the vial and began to actively use it feels much more confident. She believes that fragrance helps her become more attractive in the eyes of men, and therefore she feels less constrained, her every movement and word have her self-confidence visible and demonstrate her uniqueness. One day it will help her to find a person who will fall in love with her. And the reason for this won't be the magic fragrance, but the personal qualities of women.

Quality fragrances are still somewhat different from those used simply for the sake of a pleasant smell. Perfume with pheromones is created with the addition of such flavors, which cause the partner to feel calm and comfortable. And this is a good foundation for future family life.

The Effect of Perfume With Pheromones

Not everything that is offered by sellers, is indeed a perfume with pheromones. But quality products will still help to get at least some result. Fragrances with pheromones have their own characteristics, which are worth paying attention to.

1.   Do not expect perfume with pheromones to act as perfume water. Most often they have a rather sharp smell, which may not suit some ladies.

2.   Fragrances with pheromones have a short range. They will not attract all men who are at a distance of several meters. Attention will be paid only to those who are in close proximity.

3.   Not all men will react to that call. Modest men may not have the courage and self-confidence to approach a woman who exudes a pleasant scent and get acquainted. Some others would probably avoid this because of their girlfriend or wife. If they've got strong feelings then it usually cannot be beaten by the smell of another woman.

4.   Perfume with pheromones is not a panacea, which will help to become beloved and popular. This is just an accessory that will help emphasize other advantages. Perfume with pheromones can be regarded as a flag that attracts attention. But you still need to keep it up with the help of other advantages.

Spirits do not guarantee love, they are capable of producing only interest and sexual attraction.

5.	Care must be taken when using perfume with pheromones. No one can guarantee that they will attract only the person who you want to attract. There are also mentally unbalanced people, whose attention is not desirable. Pheromone rich fragrances can attract those people too. They might attract drunk people as well.

6.	Perfume with pheromones does not last long. It quickly erodes and ceases to function. The smell is pretty fast, the effect lasts a little longer.

7.	Such spirits do not and can not contain alcohol. It destroys pheromones.

8.	Sometimes spirits with pheromones help attract not only the opposite sex but the same sex too. This can also have its pros and cons.

9.	Perfume contains the aromas of amber and musk. Otherwise, they can not remain on the skin, combined with another flavor. Therefore, it can be noted that any perfume contains at least some pheromone part.

That's why they were commonly respected even in those times when science knew nothing about pheromones and their magic power. Perfumes with pheromones are different from the usual aromas by the number of those magical chemical elements that make it possible to attract the attention of the opposite sex.

How to Use Perfume With Pheromones the Right Way

An ancient female wisdom, derived from the quote of a great woman, says that fragrances must be applied wherever one wants to get a kiss. With some amendments, this wisdom can be applied to fragrances with pheromones.

It is necessary to put perfume so that its effect does not interfere with clothing. In addition, it will have a greater effect if it is applied to the pulsating parts of the body. Of course, the most famous are wrists. Some of it can be applied to the hollow, which is located between the clavicles. You can also put it on the elbow bend, where, if you believe perfumers, you can feel the real smell of human.

But you can spit on perfume and other parts of the body if you are planning to have a romantic evening. If the environment is intimate, and the body is not hidden by layers of clothing, then you can put some fragrance to your knee folds or ankles.

How to Buy Perfume With Pheromones

Nowadays, a large number of spirits with pheromones are produced, many of them are high quality or not that much quality fake versions. Therefore, it is worth to carefully consider the place where the perfume is going to be purchased.

It is particularly important to purchase a quality product if you take into account the price of perfume. Very rarely it is low. Some believe that the quality of the product depends on the price, but still, it is worth paying attention not only to price but also to the seller's reputation. Thanks to modern means of information, it is not that difficult to do this.

Most often, the shoppers are the internet users. You can even buy perfume directly from the manufacturers. It is still important to choose someone who can be trusted though. It is better to choose a seller who has already managed to positively recommend himself among buyers. You can read reviews and refer to those who have already purchased same or similar products.

Some sellers themselves turn to their customers, offering perfumes with pheromones at the best prices. It can be so tempting that women, forgetting about precaution, might decide to buy. But real quality perfume cannot be cheap.

Not all modern people trust internet shops. They rather prefer to buy in traditional stores. You can do this, for example, in sex shops. The shelves for adults are filled with boxes with a variety of perfumes. Still, before you go shopping, you need to turn to the Internet and read about what firms you can trust. Moreover, in adult stores, customers usually have the opportunity to try the fragrance before buying and choose the one that they like the most.

Pheromone Mystery

In any case, perfume with pheromones still remains a mystery. Pheromones and their real effect are not fully studied yet. Surprisingly, someone can manage to find the love of their whole life with the help of pheromones while others won't get much help from using it.

Each manufacturer hides the composition of his fragrances. It is believed that this helps to escape from competitors. But in the event that fragrances with pheromones are sold, such a secret can only be harmful. For example, in a bottle of perfume can be only a few drops of pheromones. So when used they will not help to get the result. Such a small amount will most likely go unnoticed. Or, there can be an alcohol in the composition of spirits, which will destroy the pheromones and make the pheromones perfume just expensive perfume water.

Others can only say that there are enough pheromones in the perfume to help them emphasize beauty, trigger the interest and lust of the opposite sex, but in fact, it is a fraud. This can be true with well-known firms too. As for their popular name, they usually earn it through the confidence that is born in the soul of a woman who uses perfume. Even if the fragrances have not produced any effect, but nevertheless the woman attracts attention at the expense of her beauty, she will still ascribe her success to the fragrances, recommend them to others and thank the creators.

Perfumes with pheromones are newcomers to the perfume market. Until now, they remain a mystery to many buyers. They are credited with special effects that help achieve the love of all the men who are around. But in fact, the effect of fragrances is somewhat different from all those rumors that grew around them.

Perfumes with pheromones help attract only those who are nearby. They begin to show attention. But this is not loving. It is only an interest and sexual attraction. The outcome of these relationships solely depends on the person. A fragrance is not able to make someone to fall in love with you, it can only attract someone to you. But, unfortunately, this applies not only to the loved ones but also to those whose attention is actually far from being desirable.

I tried and made a conclusion for myself that pheromones brought something new to me when it comes to relationships, they give confidence and affect the subconscious of person who uses them. You start to feel more confident, sexy, relaxed. This draws the attention of the people around you and the opposite sex. But do not forget that even this magical elixir cannot replace the inner qualities, spiritual beauty, and well-groomed appearance. These things can give love while perfume with pheromones can bring a sexual attraction only. Thanks to it you can become much more popular and confident.

Try and always bring something new to your life, it's exciting.

Five Female Secrets

If you are still alone or after another breakup, I want to share some more secrets with you.

After the breakup, you should spend some time alone, put your feelings in order, forget a little of the person who was part of your life. There are periods when nothing connects, but starting a new relationship does not work. Why? Have you ever wondered what the reason might be here? Is something wrong with you in this case?

The reason, in fact, is as old as the world: a girl with inflated expectations and an unreasonably high self-esteem is waiting for not just a prince, but a superhero who will turn her life into honey and a fairy tale. Of course, his ideal traits should be the same as in fashion magazines, and if not, it's torn in the pillow. Why bother yourself? Do not rush. Yes, appearance plays a role, but it is not the most important thing, do not forget about it and stop making a personality cult out of it, otherwise, you will not find the long-awaited happiness. Think and listen to yourself, it is important to feel comfortable with a person, and everything else is trifles.

Many girls experience difficulties in this aspect. Previous relationships ended, which inexorably struck on self-esteem. Do not lose yourself, continue to develop and create your life, fill it with new tasks and meaning, believe in your world and the guy who needs you will fall in love with your world. Have patience and do not forget that you need to pamper yourself.

Understand that the guy should be an important part of your life, but not the whole your life. Overcome this principle in yourself, become a self-sufficient person who knows how to appreciate life, even when you are disappointed. And most importantly - don't stop believing in love.

Men are easily fooled by standard female tricks. We neatly entangle them with our charms. Yesterday you provoked him into an acquaintance, today you are on a date, and after two months he will understand that he can not live without you. Men have their own methods of seduction, women have their own. So what are our tricks that have a magical effect on men?

1. You are the most intelligent and desired man in the world

Yes, at the beginning of a relationship woman convinces man about this, and he really feels that way. Maybe he is indeed like that, but it also can be that he only seems so, or maybe all this is just a crude flattery. But, if a man feels himself the best when he is next to you, he will strive for you, he will want to be with you more often. No doubts here.

2. I am weak and defenseless

He does not need to know how cleverly you deal with competitors, how smartly you solve conflicts, and how good you are in nailing the wall. Leave all this for now. If you want to charm him, show him that he is not only intelligent and sexy but also a strong man. And you are a defenseless being, brave but defenseless. At the same time, you are not afraid to seem weak. "How charming it is," he thinks, "how brave she is, but of course she can not cope without me."

3. Affectionate, gentle, kind

He won't escape this. You feed stray dogs, participate in charity events, or you simply gladly help those who turn to you. He knows that you are kind, disinterested, and it admires him. Still, in today's cruel world meeting such a girl is a miracle. And she is also affectionate and tender. Impressive.

4. Between obeying, and insisting on your own

A smart woman feels when she needs to agree (although she does not agree in fact) with the man, obediently, but sacrificially, nod her head and whisper: "Okay." And this will be your victory too because he will think that he won. He will first think so, and then doubt - but did I do the right thing? How can I make her happy? She's so touching, she refuses her principles and plans for me.

But there will be a time when you will do everything in your own way, and you will do it so that soon his anger will pass into silent admiration: "She is also obstinate, and not at all as simple and understandable as she seemed to me. She must be tamed, I need her."

5. Support and care

And now, when he is already falling in love with you, when you meet literally every day, you give him your love and care. You are interested in him, you take care of him, make him happy, and he does the same. But most importantly, you let him know that, in spite of your boundless love, you love yourself even more. And this will be honest.

He understands that you have already admitted him into your life, moreover, you agree to share with him everything that you have, but provided he does not try to change you if he respects your interests, your personality, if he will not own you, but love you. It is not hard to make this clear for him - just be sincere both with yourself and with him.